Healthy Eating

Making Smart Food Choices for Health and Longevity

RON KNESS

Contents

Disclaimer

We hope you enjoy reading our report however we do suggest you read our disclaimer. All the material written in this report is provided for informational purposes only and is general in nature.

Every person is a unique individual and what has worked for some or even many may not work for you. Any information perceived as advice by must be considered in light of your own particular set of circumstances.

The author or person sharing this information does not assume any responsibility for the accuracy or outcome of your use of the content.

Every attempt has been made to provide well researched and up to date content at the time of writing. Now all the legalities have been taken care of, please enjoy the content.

See your healthcare professional before starting any diet or exercise program!

Introduction

We all want to be healthy. Good health, like most things worth having, requires some effort. That effort best begins with self-education. Living a healthy lifestyle starts with what you eat. After all, "we are what we eat"!

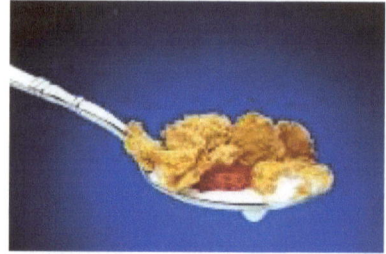

We are made personally aware of this statement when we over-indulge in poor food and drink choices. As our body deals with the consequences we feel sluggish, nauseous, irritable and lacking in energy and enthusiasm.

In modern western societies, we live in a world where our food health is usually compromised more by excess quantity than scarcity. It seems like almost all of the fast food chains have their own form of "supersizing". However, it is critical to make a distinction between sufficient or even excess food consumption and adequate nutrient intake.

In other words, more food doesn't necessarily mean it is better for you nutritionally. In fact, much of the food and drink we consume are nothing more than empty calories – calories containing very few, if any, nutrients.

The bottom line is most foods are produced with continuing and increasing sales as the major driver. How good they are for you isn't even part of the equation. To achieve this, producers and manufacturers often place more emphasis on taste, texture and appearance and shelf life rather than nutrient availability.

Good food can and does taste good, but clever processing can make foods with little nutrient value taste incredibly good too. It is up to you to know the difference and that is where this information will help you to understand why some foods and food types are better for your health, vitality and well-being. Let's get started.

What Is in the Food You Eat?

There are many foods and beverages that you may eat regularly, such as chicken nuggets, diet sodas, raspberry teas and garden burgers. However, you may not be aware that some of these foods contain added ingredients that are not food at all.

Some of these ingredients are introduced during processing to enhance taste or to act as a preservative. Many of these are dangerous or damaging to health, both physical and emotional. There is much debate and little conclusion about what are safe quantities of additives in any given food. What is a safe level for one person may be dangerous for another.

Also, the types of food that most contain artificial flavor-enhancing and preserving ingredients are those most likely to be eaten very regularly and in large amounts. These toxins may not be readily expelled by the body and the effects can be cumulative. For healthy eating, let's take a look at some ingredients you should avoid eating.

For Healthy Eating Avoid These Ingredients

Butane

Butane is certainly not just used for cigarette lighters anymore. You can also find butane in some chicken nuggets. Butane acts as an artificial antioxidant that food manufacturers use to keep chicken nuggets fresh.

Butane is also present in other frozen and packaged foods such as crackers, cereal bars and chips. So, the next time you're craving for some chicken nuggets, perhaps you might like to make some homemade ones.

Propylene Glycol

This substance is what makes your ice cream creamy and smooth, but propylene glycol is exactly the same substance used in cosmetics, deodorant and cars.

Propylene glycol is an anti-freeze substance, so be wary of this antifreeze chemical when buying cake mixes, low-fat ice creams, dog food and salad dressings.

Although it is definitely good for your vehicle, it isn't as good for your health.

Potassium Benzoate

Many people love drinking diet sodas as they want to quench their thirst whilst not drinking a lot of sugary calories. A diet soda is certainly sweet and bubbly yet it is also an unhealthy concoction.

Diet sodas can contain potassium benzoate and when ingested this can form into benzene which is a carcinogen. It can also be found in some fruit juices which contain ascorbic acid and vitamin C, and that can worsen the effects of benzene in the body.

Additionally, this substance is present in low-fat salad dressings, olives, syrups, apple cider and jams. So read your labels before purchasing.

Soy

Artificial additives are not the only ingredients to be wary of. Soy was once the darling of the health food world and touted as a replacement for many foods. Many people believe that eating soy food products for obtaining protein in their diet, is the healthiest alternative to eating meat proteins.

Recent studies are disputing this and claiming that excess soy consumption can be bad for health, and more specifically, that only some soy is actually beneficial for humans.

These studies reveal that soy is linked to problems with fertility, low estrogen levels in women and early puberty among children. Soy was also found to contribute to an imbalance of omega-3 and omega-6 fatty acids in the body.

Most of the accusations point to unfermented soy and there is increasing guidance to only consuming products made from fermented soy, preferably organic.

Avoid soy oil, soy sauce, soy milk, soy protein and soy isolate, unless they have been fermented. Currently 60% of soy and other soy-containing food products found in the market are not the fermented type.

Read the Label

Knowing about the existence of these unhealthy ingredients in our foods is a first step towards making your diet a healthier one. The biggest step is applying that knowledge – read the labels and leave the artificial additives on the shelf, especially where a more natural option is available.

To improve your family's dietary health, avoid packaged or processed foods as much as possible. Opt for natural, fresh and whole foods; try to get organic is you can.

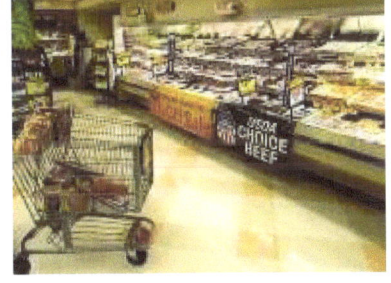

You may find it hard to forego ice cream or diet sodas, but once you get used to NOT having them, you will find that you will actually lose the cravings for many unhealthy fast and processed foods.

Healthy food selection, like all good habits, is one certainly worth developing.

Healthy Lifestyle Diets

The road towards optimum health and longevity starts with, and continually depends upon, good nutrition. If you want a healthy mind and body, you need to follow a healthy lifestyle diet plan. The bottom line is the single biggest factor to our health, or lack of, that we have the most personal control over, is the food we eat.

All too often, as we unmindfully seek out tastier and tastier eating options, we let our taste buds rather than our thinking minds choose our food for us. These are not necessarily the best choices for our health, especially over the long term.

Even when you do decide to make conscious, healthy eating choices, you will be faced with an overwhelming array of "healthy" options, each with its own band of advocates and detractors.

Although some diets can be described as 'fad' 'extreme' or even 'dangerous', there are still many other more mainstream diets that appear to be in direct conflict with each other.

The main reason for this is that diets are not one-size-fits-all. What works for one person may not work for another. Different diets call for different levels of willpower, inclusions and exclusions. Some are based on blood type and ancestry.

While it is not in anyone's best interest to jump from one diet to another testing them all, it can be very worthwhile researching which diet style is best for you, based on all your known factors, especially lifestyle.

One type of healthy lifestyle diet that has been proven to provide many health benefits is the low-fat, high-fiber diet.

There are many cases of gastrointestinal problems which have been resolved after following a low-fat, high-fiber diet plan. For those who have colorectal cancer, this diet has been used to reduce and lessen the chances of the cancer recurring.

A low-fat, high-fiber diet can also be an important part of a treatment plan for people who are suffering from hemorrhoids, constipation and diverticulitis. Those diagnosed with cardiovascular disease may greatly help prevent the condition from getting worse if they increase their fiber and reduce their fat intake.

If you are diabetic or simply want to lose weight, this kind of diet plan can also be very beneficial. Foods that contain low levels of fat tend to be low in calories, thereby reducing the risk of obesity and other diseases associated with being over-weight.

Low-Fat Food Choices

A low-fat diet does not have to be either bland or tasteless.

With a little planning you can build an enjoyable low-fat, high-fiber diet plan around:

- Legumes

- Whole Grain Foods

- Fruits and Vegetables

Legumes

Legumes are excellent replacements for refined carbohydrates. Legumes are great sources of fiber, calcium, protein, vitamins and minerals and they help prevent food cravings and metabolic syndrome.

Eating legumes instead of refined carbohydrates will make it easier to maintain stable blood sugar levels. Legumes are helpful for the proper functioning of the pancreas and help prevent the pancreas from producing too much insulin.

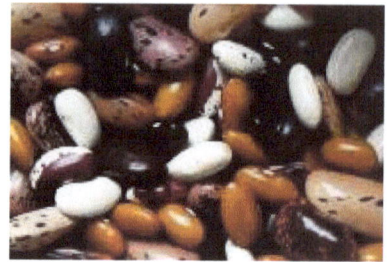

Examples of legumes, include beans, garbanzo, lentils and peas. Mixing these different legumes in your soups, burritos and salad recipes will add variety to your daily diet.

Whole Grain

Whole grains have a much higher fiber content than refined grains. They are also rich in B vitamins, antioxidants and other important trace minerals (i.e. copper, iron, magnesium and zinc).

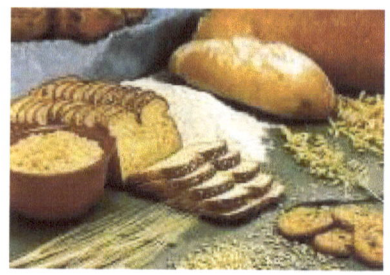

These foods are crucial for the growth of healthy bacteria in the colon while improving overall bowel health at the same time.

Whole grain corn, bulgur, whole rye, quinoa, sorghum, brown rice and buckwheat are a few examples of whole grain foods.

Avoid buying foods that are labeled with the words "cracked wheat", "stone-ground" and "multi-grain". These labels suggest that they are not whole grain foods. Make sure to read the labels well before finally making that purchase.

Fruits and Vegetables

Fruits and vegetables generally contain soluble fiber which can help you reduce your levels of the bad LDL cholesterol.

Broccoli, kale, zucchini, dark lettuce, cauliflower and other green leafy vegetables are good sources of high fiber. Others are raspberries, grapefruit, mango, bananas, oranges and plums.

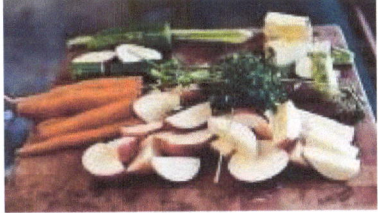

Your meals do not have to be boring because there are plenty of recipes that you can make. Add variety to your daily diet as much as possible and look for ingredients and cooking instructions for great tasting low fat, high fiber recipes.

Carbohydrates In Your Diet

Breads, sugars and pastas are all carbohydrate foods and are the staples of many people's diets. Carbohydrates have been receiving a bad reputation in the past few years. Unfortunately, lumping all carbs into the 'bad' basket has caused much confusion and disinformation for those concerned about their nutrition.

There was a time, not too long ago, when all fats were considered bad. Longer term studies have shown convincingly that some dietary fat is very beneficial and necessary to human health. There are good fats and bad fats. There is good cholesterol and bad cholesterol. Similarly, there are carbohydrates which, when not eaten to excess, are good for us. Others are not so good, or even unhealthy.

Some carb sources have been highly regarded as being very helpful for the prevention of some chronic diseases.

This brings us to a commonly asked question, 'which carbs are good and which carbs are bad?'

The Good Carbohydrates

Complex carbohydrates are considered good carbs because they provide the body with a useable source of energy as well as fiber and other dietary nutrients in addition to the carbohydrate content. The carbohydrate is slowly broken down by the body into glucose. These are the types of carbs that keep our blood sugar levels steady all throughout the day, without making us experience hunger pangs.

Unlike simple carbs, complex carbohydrates also reduce the prevalence of mood swings and reduce the likelihood of feeling irritable.

Examples of good carbohydrate foods include whole meal pasta, brown rice, potatoes, whole grains, legumes, beans, peas and nuts. It also includes dairy products that are not processed with added sugar.

The Bad Carbohydrates

Bad carbohydrates are those foods that are referred to as simple carbohydrates. These are the types of carbs that are broken down by the body too rapidly for the body to use the released glucose. If left in the bloodstream, this excess is dangerous to parts of the body such as the eyes, so the body moves quickly to sweep it into body tissues and organs. The excess is mostly stored as unwanted and unhealthy body fat.

Simple carbohydrates are found in foods that are made from refined sugar and processed flours such as cakes, cookies, soft drinks, chips and alcoholic beverages. It also includes white rice and food made largely from white flour, including many pasta types.

These foods are digested by the body very quickly, so they cause people to experience blood sugar 'spikes'. These spikes are what causes you to have an energy crash. Eating too many bad carbohydrates may over time increase the risk of heart diseases and diabetes.

The Importance of Carbohydrates

Glucose is the unit of sugar that the body uses as one of its sources of energy. Moderate amounts of complex carbohydrates are effective suppliers of glucose while also supplying vitamins, minerals and fiber.

The problem arises when we eat only simple carbs regularly and in large quantities. It is one of the biggest reasons for our obesity problem of today. Too many soft drinks, cakes, donuts and fried foods are coated with more carbs.

Excess simple carb consumption leads to excess stored body fat.

In order to meet the body's daily nutritional requirement, adults in a healthy weight range can obtain 45-65 per cent of calories from their carbohydrate intake. Those wanting to reduce unwanted fat can replace some of these carbs with protein to lose weight without restricting their calorie intake.

It makes good dietary sense to choose to eat good complex carbs instead of simple carbs to make up the carbohydrate component of your diet.

Along with your carbs, eat plenty of protein rich foods that are also sources of other needed vitamins, minerals and nutrients. A healthy, balanced diet lowers your risk of many lifestyle diseases.

Genetically Modified Foods and Your Health

GMO's or Genetically Modified Organisms refer to living things, usually food crops, that have undergone a process of gene material altering. DNA is taken from one species and artificially inserted into the genes of another species, such as an unrelated flora or fauna species.

This process creates a new species. The claimed benefits of this process include disease and pest resistance. While this might sound like something out of a Frankenstein laboratory, humans are very clever and have done some amazing things over time, both good and bad.

There are many claims and counter-claims regarding genetically modified food.

Big Companies, Big Dollars at Stake

One huge corporation is responsible for most of the advances in this field.

They spend a large amount of money to support their claims that their genetic modifications will help feed a hungry world, by helping farmers grow bounteous crops, more easily.

However, it does not take much research to be at least a bit cynical of their claims, and that their main goal is making money. The very heart of the matter is that every time a plant is genetically modified, the newly created plant is patented by the creating company.

Patents on Life

They own the rights to the plants and its seeds. Part of the conditions of purchase of any seed is that the new owner is not allowed to harvest or regrow seed obtained from them.

All seed must be purchased anew for the next season's crop. If seed is retained and sown the company will sue the farmer.

This company has lobbied governments to change their laws to the extent that even when seed has blown onto a neighboring farmer's land, and naturally re-sown, that farmer has been successfully sued for growing the patented DNA product.

Many people believe that allowing a corporation to have patents over living organisms is evil. While the legal and moral implications of GMO's continue to be debated and argued in courts of law, for most of us the burning question is are they safe for us to eat?

Strong claims from both sides mean the consumer is no clearer as to the health implications of consuming these foods. One problem is that there is little financial support or incentive for long term studies which may prove that there are health problems associated with GMO's.

The money is strongly stacked on the other side. Fears have been expressed by knowledgeable scientists and researchers that there is a very real possibility of future damage to human health due to long term consumption of these foods.

Claims include reduced nutrient value as compared to unmodified equivalents. More frightening are claims that these altered genes could trigger changes in our own DNA, not discernable in ourselves, that may be passed to our offspring.

Studies which have been done on other animals have shown reduced fertility when fed large amounts of certain GMO foods. A real concern is that the non-food genes introduced into food could cause severe allergen responses in humans, as our bodies react to a perceived threat.

As much of the genetic engineering attempts to create crops which are resistant to pests, there is a fear that whatever genes are included to kill or resist pests, it could be dangerous to humans over time in large amounts.

Lifetime Effects

Long term antibiotic resistance is also considered a real possibility; as genetic engineers rely heavily on the use of antibiotics when conducting their experiments.

Genetically modified foods are becoming more prevalent, especially with some major food staples. In some countries there are a few crops that are almost unavailable as non-GM.

There are no health benefits of eating GMO food. Because there is so much uncertainty and misinformation about GMO foods, many are choosing to totally shun them.

Given the potential downside for long term human health, this would seem to be the wisest choice.

The Safest Option?

In the future, if somehow GMO foods prove to be non-damaging, you will have lost nothing by having not eaten them. On the other hand, if they do prove dangerous, and you have been consuming them, you will not be able to undo the effects on yourself and perhaps even your offspring.

This is where the old saying "an ounce of prevention is better than a pound of cure" best applies. As much as possible, prevent these foods from being consumed by not buying them in your weekly grocery shopping. Knowledge will serve 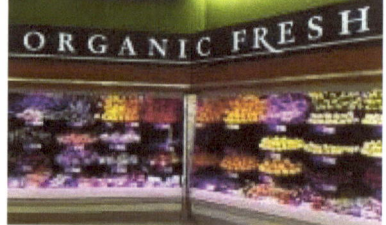 as your best weapon against GM foods. You should check the foods you are buying and assess whether the food comes from a non-GMO source.

Stay Informed

More information you need to make your choices can easily be found on the Internet. Be a wise consumer and start by being a well-informed one.

Health Problems in Eating Grains

Many people suffer with health problems after eating foods made from grain. You may be someone who does too and perhaps you don't know the real reason why. Here are some of the substances contained in grains that are known to cause problems.

Gluten

Wheat consumed today is entirely different to the wheat 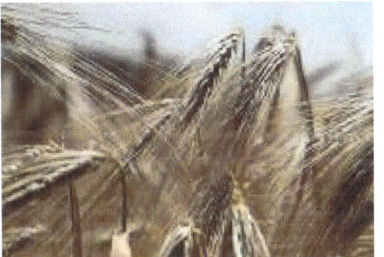 consumed centuries ago. The wheat produced today for human consumption has been aggressively hybridized and crossbred. As the wheat has become genetically tweaked its gluten content has also increased up to as much as 50%.

Gluten is not easy for humans to digest which means that once consumed, your body has extra strain put on your digestive system.

Gluten consumption can increase the permeability of your intestines which can lead to leaky gut syndrome. Leaky gut syndrome is a loosely-defined condition which can have differing causes and is not even recognized as a real condition by some doctors. If it occurs, dietary components that are not yet completely digested may enter your bloodstream, resulting in several health issues.

There are about 55 diseases which have been associated with gluten consumption. Gluten consumption can increase your risk of inflammatory bowel disease, anemia, osteoporosis, canker sores, rheumatoid arthritis and many other autoimmune diseases.

There are also studies that link gluten consumption to several psychiatric and neurological diseases such as depression, anxiety, migraines, epilepsy, neuropathy and dementia.

Phytic Acid

Phytic acid is usually found in the bran of grains and has been known to block the absorption of minerals, such as magnesium, iron, zinc, copper and calcium.

People who consume large amounts of grain-based foods are at higher risk of bone-related illnesses such as osteoporosis because of the mineral suppression that occurs.

One way to avoid this problem is by letting the grains sprout before using them. It is through 'sprouting' that the grains are able to break down their phytic acid content and make their mineral content available.

Lectins

In addition to gluten and phytic acid, grains may also contain lectins that are sugar-binding proteins. In plants, lectins function as natural defenders to protect the plants against parasites and molds. Each time the plant senses any attack from these invaders they counter-attack by immediately binding to the foreign sugar molecules they contain.

However, when these lectins make their way into your digestive system, they do the same thing against sugar molecules in your system. Unfortunately, this can have a harmful effect because the lining of the digestive system has sugar-containing cells that are crucial for breaking down food.

When lectins attack those sugar containing cells in your digestive system, your immune system retaliates. Our body's digestive enzymes cannot alter lectins, so our gut permeability may be altered.

Once these lectins penetrate the bloodstream they then bind to any tissues found in the pancreas or thyroid. This act of binding can disrupt the functioning of the tissues triggering a counter-attack from the white blood cells.

In simple terms, eating grains that contain lectins can set off a chain reaction of an autoimmune response. This explains why so many degenerative and chronic inflammatory diseases are endemic to populations who regularly consume wheat and wheat-based foods.

These lectins may be small, but they are designed by nature to be resistant to any attacks by other living systems so they cannot be broken down. They continue to accumulate until they bind into the tissues and cause interference in many biological processes that are taking place inside our body.

As grains are relatively easy to grow in large volumes, they have become an increasingly larger portion of our overall diet. As well as being the major ingredient of many staple foods, they are also used as fillers in many others.

It can be surprisingly difficult to eradicate grains from a modern diet, but if you are suffering from dietary upsets, simply reducing your macro grain sources, such as bread and pasta, may give quick relief.

Eating Whole Grains and Reducing Cancer Risks

On the contrary to the potential problems of eating refined grains, whole grains can be good for you ... especially when it comes to the prevention of cancer. An increased consumption of whole grains has been found by some studies to greatly reduce one's risk for developing cancer. Many people do eat whole grains and those who follow the macrobiotic diet, eat a diet that consists of 50-60% of whole grains. Some of these grains include buckwheat, brown rice, quinoa, lentils, corn and rye.

Whole Grains as Good Sources of Fiber

Several studies showed that an increased consumption of whole grains can help reduce the risk for developing colorectal cancer.

This is made possible due to the high fiber content adding bulk to the digestive system, which speed up the digestive process and reduces the length of time that it takes for food wastes to travel into and through the colon.

This shortened-travel time is beneficial, especially if the food waste contains carcinogens as they need to be removed from the body as quickly as possible. As a result, the risk of the lower intestines being affected by these carcinogens will be greatly reduced.

In addition, as fiber is broken down in the lower intestine with the help of bacteria, a substance called butyrate is also produced. Butyrate is known to be helpful for inhibiting the growth of certain types of cancer such as rectum and colon cancer.

Fiber Binds to Estrogen

The dietary fiber found in whole grains also plays a key role in the prevention of breast cancer. This is because fiber has the capability of binding to estrogen.

Having excess levels of estrogen in the body is known to increase the risk of breast cancer. Regular consumption of whole grains helps the liver to filter out estrogen from the bloodstream. Fiber helps expedite the process of removing excess estrogens and prevents them from causing the body harm, thereby helping reduce the risk of developing breast cancer.

Whole Grains Contain Selenium

Several studies have shown that a selenium deficiency can increase the likelihood of several types of cancers developing. The amount of selenium obtained from the grains varies depending on the selenium content of the soil where the grains are grown. An adequate intake of selenium obtained from dietary sources was found to significantly reduce the risk of colorectal and prostate cancers. These types of cancers are two of the most common types of cancer.

A clinical trial showed that a 200mg dose of selenium daily can reduce cancer by as much as 37%. Test tube studies showed that selenium inhibits the growth of tumors and helps ensure that cells die before they become malignant. Selenium is also found to work in synergy with vitamin E in preventing the formation of carcinogens. Another reason why selenium reduces the risk of cancer is because it has the ability to activate a specific enzyme which is responsible for preventing the formation of free radicals.

Grain and Your Insulin Levels

Other studies have shown that the increased consumption of whole grains can help reduce an individual's insulin levels. Having excess levels of serum insulin can increase the risk for breast, colon and other cancers.

The list of cancer reducing benefits that you can obtain by eating whole grains is quite substantial, especially when whole grains replace highly refined grains in the diet. Individuals need to test their own reactions to a high grain diet, even when whole grain is use, as some people's systems cannot tolerate high grain consumption.

Diet and Cancer

Not too long ago, within living memory of those now consider aged, cancer did occur, but at nowhere near the rate seen today. The last few generations have seen such an explosion in diagnoses of cancer that people describe it as a cancer epidemic, even though cancer is not contagious. For many of those who have lost a loved one to cancer, their greatest fear is contracting some form of cancer themselves and they live a life of dread between doctors' visits.

Worldwide, billions are spent annually on cancer research. Researchers look for causes, triggers, clusters, and commonality. They test drugs, foods and other methods to reduce or remove tumor growth.

Those who lack medical knowledge talk hopefully of a "cure for cancer", as if one day there will be either a surgical procedure or a pharmaceutical product that will magically stop and reverse all the different types of cancer. Many people have overcome cancer; they usually speak of being in remission, rather than cured; hopefully the remission will last the rest of their lives.

Diet and Cancer

Researchers crunch the data to discover a common theme or cause for the exponential increase in cancer incidence. They are finding in step, a change of diet in those societies where cancer is increasing. In so-called advanced societies, over the last eighty years or so, diets have changed dramatically.

What is also entering public consciousness is that the increasing incidence of cancer may also be related to these changes in diet. This does not necessarily mean that diet is the cause of cancer, as the likelihood of contracting cancer may be greatly influenced by genetics and environmental causes. However, most non-accident maladies have components of both breeding (genetic pre-disposition) and feeding (environmental and dietary influences).

Where once a big health risk was malnutrition or starvation from a lack of food, today it is more likely a malnutrition caused by the overconsumption of poor dietary choices that is causing a raft of lifestyle diseases.

A normal diet of rationed servings of mainly vegetables and meat (complex carbs, protein and meat-derived fat) with plain water as the main or only drink has morphed into a normal diet of very large servings of an incredible variety of pre-cooked and processed foods.

Today, every day, in addition to eating some highly processed meat and maybe some vegetables, often containing taste enhancers such as sauces, crumbing, etc. (simple carbs and modified vegetable fats) most people also consume desserts (simple carbs), snacks (simple carbs) with soft drink (more simple carbs) as their main fluid source.

Dietary Links to Lifestyle Diseases

There are indisputable parallels in the dietary changes and the health problems in western societies. Obesity, type two diabetes and cancer appear more commonly to be linked not only to one another, but to diet. Data studies prove that increased cancer incidence is linked to obesity. If type two diabetes is confirmed the incidence is even higher.

Observations of indigenous societies and those who have maintained traditional diets show no noticeable increase in markers for these diseases. Where western influences have changed the diets of others, their disease rates have exploded within a single generation. There is an incredibly strong correlation between diet and the incidence of cancer, as well as diabetes and obesity.

The Future and You

Relevant studies are ongoing, but research costs money and the big money is to be made in the production, sale and promotion of foods that are based on taste and therefore repeat sales rather than health. Cancer is a disease where prevention is thousands of time better than a cure, as anyone who has dealt with cancer can affirm.

Even if the weight of non-dietary factors is against you, you have the power to massively reduce your likelihood of succumbing to cancer by taking positive control over the food you eat. Anyone who is concerned about avoiding cancer should take steps to largely eliminate simple sugar foods and highly processed foods from their diet. There are plenty of healthy unrefined choices available as replacements.

Eating Healthy to Prevent Macular Degeneration

Did you know you can help prevent macular degeneration by eating healthy?

Macular degeneration is one of the most common causes of blindness in mature people and is known as AMD – Age Related Macular Degeneration.

It is a condition that damages an individual's central vision. The central vision is the part of the eye that is mostly responsible for your vision when reading or driving. It is the same part of the eye that is used for seeing fine details.

Although macular degeneration does not cause any pain, it can eventually lead to blindness.

Did you know that your diet can play a large part in lowering or worsening your risk of developing macular degeneration?

To help prevent it, you can start eating healthier now.

Beta-Carotene, Vitamins C and E

Researchers in the Netherlands conducted a study which was aimed at finding how a person's diet can affect their risk of developing macular degeneration. The study conducted was over an 8-year period, consisting of 4,000 people.

It was found that those in the study who ate plenty of foods rich in beta-carotene and vitamins C and E, lowered their risks of developing macular degeneration by up to 35%. Those whose diet was not as healthy or nutritious as the average, had a 20% increased risk of developing macular degeneration.

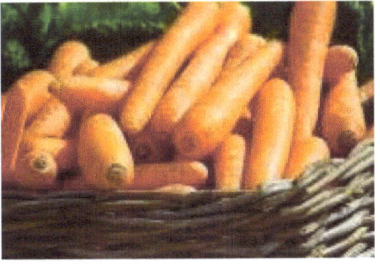

Zinc

Eating foods that contain zinc, or zinc supplements will also be beneficial to eye health. The retina contains zinc which plays a crucial role in the proper functioning of eye enzymes. Those afflicted with AMD have very low levels of zinc in the retina.

Zeaxanthin and Lutein – Inseparable Antioxidants

Foods which contain lutein also contain the antioxidant zeaxanthin. Experts have found that the tissues of the macula have high concentrations of these paired antioxidants. As much as 90% of blue light that enters the eyes are being absorbed by the macula and these antioxidants function as a sunscreen to filter out the damaging rays.

Our bodies do not have the capability to produce these kinds of antioxidants, so we need to obtain them from our daily diet.

Foods such as broccoli, Romaine lettuce, collards, spinach and kale are known to be helpful in increasing the pigment density in a person's macula.

Greater pigment density in the macula means higher levels of protection for the retina which may additionally translate to lowered risks of macular degeneration and cataract formation.

Omega-3 Fatty Acids

Omega-3 fatty acids increase protection for the light receptor cells in a person's eyes. Having high levels of omega 3 fatty acids helps protect the eyes from damage which can be caused by free radicals and too much exposure to sunlight.

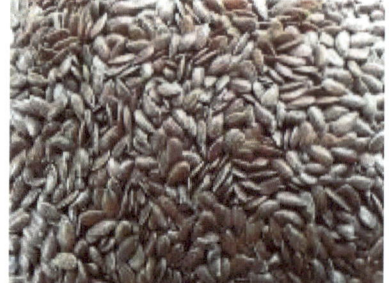

Eating one serving daily of omega-3-rich foods, such as salmon, walnuts, flax seeds or beans, can help lower one's risk of macular degeneration by up to 30%.

A study showed that regular consumption of foods rich in omega-3 fatty acids helped those people who had early signs of AMD and reduced their risk of advanced symptoms.

Avoid Sugar

It is equally important to note that eating sugary foods and those that are made from refined starch can be detrimental to eye health. These low-quality, low-nutrient carbohydrate foods can increase the risks of getting cataracts and AMD.

Low-quality carbs have a high glycemic index which can lead to having high sugar concentrations in the eyes. Frequent and long-term consumption of sugary foods can cause inflammation and oxidative stress which may eventually damage the tiny capillaries and the retina in the eyes.

Increasing your consumption of the foods high in nutrients and minimizing your intake of foods that contain low-quality carbs will help to prevent macular degeneration.

Do You Drink Too Much Coffee?

For many people, a cup of coffee is an indispensable part of their morning routine and more often than not, there are many other perfect times for that next indispensable cup too!

While coffee may seem to be helpful in keeping you awake and alert, too much of a good thing can be damaging to your health. It is recommended to limit your coffee intake in order to avoid caffeine-related health problems. Be self-aware enough to watch for signs that your coffee habit may be affecting your health.

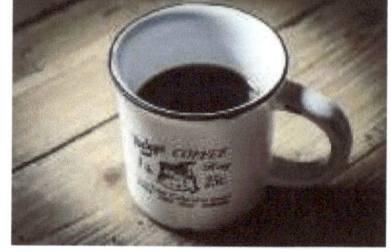

Experiment with drinking less coffee or switching to decaf, if only to monitor for signs of addiction to caffeine.

Do you have dark colored urine?

Having orange colored or dark colored urine, if you have not been engaged in physical activity, is one sign that you may have been drinking too many caffeine beverages.

When your urine is yellow or orange in color, then your body is becoming dehydrated.

Caffeine is a diuretic, so if you want to avoid dehydration, limit your coffee intake to two cups in a day. If you have more, don't consider your coffee as part of your fluid intake. Drink a couple of extra glasses of water to replace lost fluids.

Do you suffer with frequent headaches?

Caffeine can trigger migraine attacks because of the effect of the stimulant on the brain. If you find yourself having frequent headaches, try cutting back on your caffeine intake and see if you experience positive results.

Headaches can also be the result of not being able to get enough quality sleep at night which can also be caused by drinking too much caffeine during the day. Even if you love your morning coffee, switch to tea or water in the afternoon.

Do you find it hard to sleep at night?

If it takes you thirty minutes or more to fall asleep at night, then you should consider reducing your caffeine intake. This is because caffeine can remain in the body for eight to fourteen hours which means it can have adverse effects on your sleeping hours even if drunk much earlier.

To help with falling asleep easier, avoid drinking coffee and any caffeinated beverages after lunch. The effects of sleep loss and sleep deprivation can accumulate into a bigger problem over time.

It can negatively affect your daily performance, leading to reduced productivity levels and decline in your overall health.

Do you experience anxiety?

Are you someone who suffers with anxiety or related problems? If so, caffeine can exacerbate your anxiety symptoms. Even if you do not have an anxiety problem, drinking too much caffeine can lead to the same symptoms experienced with anxiety, such as rapid heartbeat, sweaty palms and restlessness.

It is certainly not in your best interest to have a cup of coffee if you are already feeling anxious as your agitation will increase. Have an herbal tea, such as chamomile, instead.

Experiencing muscle tremors is another tell-tale sign of overdosing on caffeine, which can also further exacerbate one's anxiety. Muscle tremors can occur because caffeine has the tendency to over stimulate the nervous system.

This is due to caffeine causing adverse effects on the tranquilizing neurotransmitter chemicals known as adenosine.

The stimulant effects of caffeine also trigger the production of adrenaline thereby making an individual experience worsened anxiety symptoms.

Severe cases of excess consumption of caffeine have been often linked to cases of depression, but this may be a symptom as well as a cause.

How your body responds to caffeine can largely depend on how much your body is conditioned to having it. People who are not used to drinking coffee on a regular basis tend to be more sensitive to its effects.

As with alcohol, the same is true for coffee - drink in moderation to avoid possible impacts on your health, now and in the future.

Food Cravings

Food cravings - we almost all experience them at some time or another. Some people are lucky enough to be strong enough to resist their cravings. However, many find it hard to resist their cravings and end up suffering from obesity and other serious health problems as a result.

Our food cravings don't necessarily mean we are hungry; it is often our brain that has triggered the want or need for specific types of foods. Unfortunately, this response is governed not by the thinking part of our brain, but by the part that controls instinct and survival.

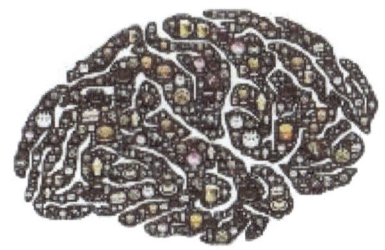

The brain's response to a perceived lack will trigger hunger symptoms. These may be specific (for a particular food or food type) or non-specific, but this primitive urge is focused on instant satisfaction rather than mindful evaluation as to best dietary choices. It is up to each of us to pause and make conscious, considered decisions about each food item we eat.

Craving Salty Foods

People who try to cut salty foods from their diet will very likely experience cravings for those same foods as the body rebalances its mineral makeup. This is especially true if you have been accustomed to eating salty foods for many years.

Craving salty food is usually based on habit and the conditioning of our taste buds, however in some cases, it is possible that a medical reason may exist, such as a trace mineral deficiency. A lack of specific minerals that contribute to our electrolyte make-up can 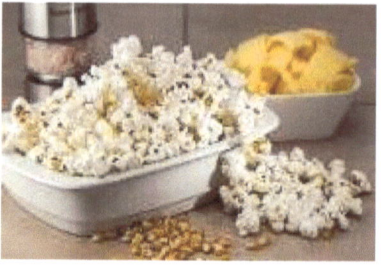 cause us to seek any source of salt. Unfortunately, common table salt is only potassium chloride and the needed minerals may not be provided by it.

Craving salt could also be a result of stress hormone fluctuations in the body. It is obviously much better to find healthier ways to reduce stress instead of snacking.

Even though in the short term your adrenal glands will help you cope with these stressors, they can become fatigued from dealing with a constant increase of producing stress hormones.

Chronic adrenal fatigue can cause a raft of other problems and can take years to repair. Adrenal glands that have become exhausted may benefit from a diet rich in green leafy vegetables. This can help them replenish their supply of potassium and other trace minerals.

Studies have revealed that taking the time to meditate and indulge in other relaxation exercises can help lower one's cravings for salty foods by as much as 25 percent.

Another possible reason for salty food cravings is dehydration. Frequent perspiration during hot weather or after exercise may lead you to lose excessive amounts of electrolytes.

In very rare cases, people who crave salty foods have been diagnosed with a serious medical condition known as hypoparathyroidism.

Craving Chocolate

Chocolate contains an antidepressant that is commonly craved by people who wish to have a quick 'pick-me-up' after a gloomy day. The improvement in mood can be attributed to the tryptophan content in chocolate. Tryptophan is an amino acid that is essential for serotonin production.

One of the reasons people crave chocolate is because their bodies lack serotonin. If a person has low serotonin levels in the brain, they may feel dissatisfied and stressed. However, once chocolate is consumed their serotonin levels increase and this typically makes them feel happier and 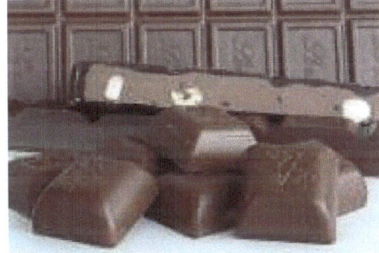 balances their mood, at least in the short term.

A deficiency in the macro mineral magnesium is also another reason for chocolate cravings. Chocolate is rich in magnesium. If you want to enjoy a tasty source of magnesium, try eating raw chocolate or cocoa powder.

Craving Spicy Foods

Spicy foods can trigger immediate perspiration. This explains the seemingly strange behavior whereby some people crave spicy foods when the weather becomes too hot for them to handle. The more they eat spicy foods, the more they sweat, preventing their body from overheating further.

Some people however, simply crave spicy foods because they have become addicted to the 'spicy thrill' that occurs. This can cause an increased heart rate and rapid breathing.

Craving Sweets

Many individuals gravitate towards sweets as comfort foods.

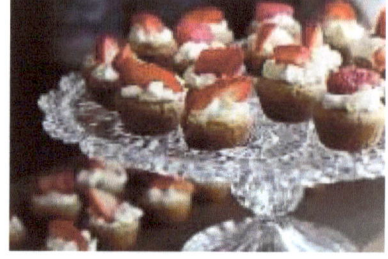

This can be in response to fluctuations in blood sugar levels, often caused by a previous binge on simple carbohydrate foods and the subsequent insulin release. This causes sub-normal blood sugar levels, leading to fatigue and feelings of ill-mood or depression.

If this situation becomes frequent and chronic, it is possible that you may end up dealing with hypoglycemia. This means that your body may experience low and potentially dangerous levels of blood sugar.

Instead of choosing sweets that are loaded with simple sugars, carbohydrates and empty calories, it would be more beneficial to enjoy some whole fruit to satisfy your cravings for sweet foods.

Even though the majority of us experience food cravings, it does not mean that it is necessarily healthy to succumb to them. If your food cravings are left unmanaged, it can easily lead to repetitive gorging or binge-eating patterns. This can result in long-term health problems such as obesity, diabetes and other diseases.

Final Thoughts

The fight against ill-health and many diseases starts with eating a healthy diet. So many modern medical cures are really attempts to undo the damage caused by poor dietary choices.

Of course there are people who can't eat healthy foods due to their circumstances, either environmental or financial. Too often though, lack of finance is given as an excuse for not eating healthy foods. Way too often the real culprits are:

Not taking the time to educate one's self about real nutrient requirements.

Letting taste buds define food choices.

Taking the easy, convenient, processed option.

This is mainly because processed foods are readily accessible and just as prevalent, or more so, as healthy food choices. The trouble lies in trying to resist the ease and convenience that fast foods provide and this is the root cause of so many health problems.

A healthy diet really should be the number one priority in a person's life so that a healthy mind and body happens automatically! If the mind is healthy, happy relationships can form. If the body is healthy, disease has a harder time to set in. If the mind and body are both healthy all good things are possible, and certainly far more likely.

Weight Management

This is self-evident. A healthy balanced diet makes managing your weight easy. For people wanting to win against the battle of obesity, a good start is to cut back on high carbohydrate content food.

Make good dietary choices a lifestyle, not a short-term fix. You are in this for life! Go for a diet that is lower in calories but high in nutrients. Eat some fruit and increase vegetable consumption. Animal meat and poultry products provide excellent protein, but eat them as close to natural as possible, don't lather them with sauces and crumb coatings. Stay away from foods that contain simple carbohydrates such as white bread, pastries, cakes and candies.

More Energy

Our diet must provide the right amount and type of nutrients containing good calories for us to have enough energy. This energy will be used by the body so that thought, healing and growth processes will be able to function properly. Healthy foods greatly improve performance, alertness and brain health.

Prevent Diseases

Failure to observe a healthy diet puts anyone at a higher risk of heart disease, diabetes, cancer and other serious illnesses. Your diet should not contain too many foods that are high in saturated and trans fats, as these are known to be linked to an increased incidence of stroke and heart attack.

Saturated and trans fats can be found in cookies, vegetable shortenings, some margarines and any other foods that are fried using partially hydrogenated oils. Trans fats increase your risk of coronary heart diseases. Use olive oil when cooking and if using margarine choose one made from olive oil too.

Improve Mood

The right foods can do wonders in improving your mood. However, do not succumb to emotional eating. Emotion-driven food binges will almost certainly be poor dietary choices and the effects will be very temporary – leading to repeated bad patterns of behavior.

Foods that contain important nutrients such as vitamin B folate help in combating anxiety and depression. Foods that are rich in B vitamins help in the production of serotonin in the brain. Serotonin is a neurotransmitter that can affect behavior and moods.

Better Mental Performance

Studies have shown that people who eat foods that are rich in vitamins B, C, D and E, plus omega-3 fatty acids have better performance in several cognitive tests compared to those who did not eat fruits, vegetables and fish.

Researchers are providing more and more evidence that having a healthy diet will help prevent diseases related to brain-shrinkage.

Take Control of Your Food Choices

Make a lifelong habit of basing your daily food intake on mindful healthy choices. This will help avoid developing many of the lifestyle illnesses that will cause ongoing health problems in your life.

There are far more food choices on offer than most of us need. In most cases, mindful eating comes down to what we don't eat – that is, avoiding foods that we know aren't good for us. There are plenty of foods that are both tasty and healthy.

Other Health and Fitness Books by This Author

If you would like to read more about Health and Fitness, here is a list of the titles, CreateSpace links and descriptions:

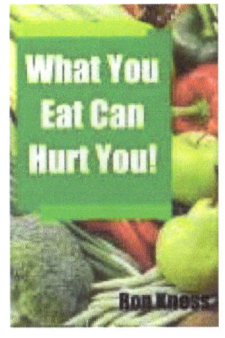

What You Eat Can Hurt You

https://www.createspace.com/4963196

Do you know that certain foods increase your risk for inflammation, disease and illness? It's true! And certain foods can help cure and heal you if you do get sick. Knowing which foods to eat and which ones to avoid empowers you to manage your own health.

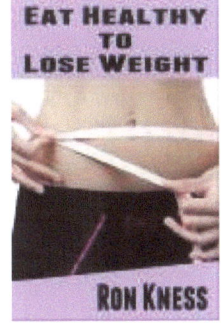

Eat Healthy to Lose Weight

https://www.createspace.com/4962939

As you read through our book, we show you which foods you should and should not be eating to reach your weight loss goal, along with discussing how to maintain your weight loss and stay within a few pounds of your goal weight. Banish the weight you keep gaining back each time by learning how to live a healthy lifestyle.

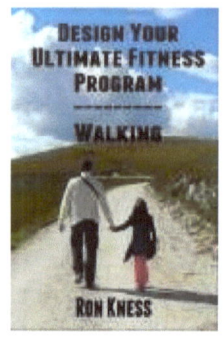

Design Your Ultimate Fitness Program - Walking

https://www.createspace.com/5252272

In my book Design Your Ultimate Fitness Program – Walking, we discuss the considerations that need to be made when designing a custom walking program, along with:
• Equipment needed
• Wearable technology you can use to track your walking
• And how to make walking more challenging

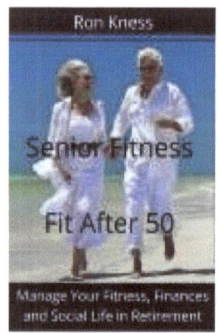

Senior Fitness – Fit After 50: Learn How to Manage Your Fitness, Finances and Social Life in Retirement

https://www.createspace.com/5474751

Inside you will discover answers to your most pressing questions:
• What do I need to know about downsizing my home?
• What are the best tips for staying healthy as you approach your 50's?
• When should I start planning for retirement?
• I am worried about being lonely once I retire, do others feel the same?
• Is it worthwhile to carry two homes during retirement?
And more…

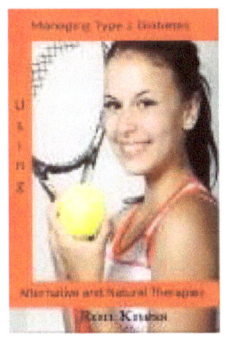

Managing Type 2 Diabetes Using Alternative And Natural Therapies

https://www.createspace.com/5401244

While Type 2 diabetes can be managed medically, there are many alternative natural and holistic methods of therapy and treatment that can further enhance quality of life and minimize the effects of this disease. In this book, I discuss 12 different types, including yoga, reflexology and acupuncture to name just three.

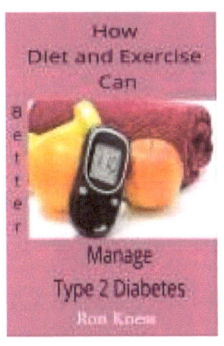

How Diet and Exercise Can Better Manage Type 2 Diabetes

https://www.crcatespace.com/5404845

Of the different types of diabetes, only Type 2 can be reversed. In my book How Diet and Exercise Can Better Manage Type 2 Diabetes, we reveal the three things you can do to best manage your disease, including:
• Diet
• Exercise
• Weight management

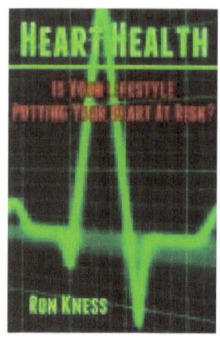

Heart Health: Is Your Lifestyle Putting Your Heart at Risk?

https://www.createspace.com/5464020

In my ebook Is Your Lifestyle Putting Your Heart At Risk? we discuss the six greatest risks to your heart and the lifestyle changes you can make to mitigate them.

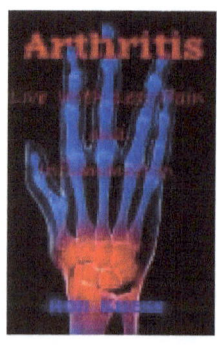

Arthritis – Live Wth Less Pain and Inflammation: Tips and Techniques You Can Use to Lessen the Pain and Inflammation

https://www.createspace.com/5457441

Discover Simple Tips & Information That Will Help Reduce The Painful Symptoms Of Arthritis!

You learn things like:
• Simple and effective information that will help you manage the pain and inflammation that comes along with arthritis, so that you can live an active, full life without debilitating pain.
• The different types of arthritis, their symptoms and how to alleviate their painful side effects.
• The pros and cons of over-the-counter arthritis medications, plus simple tips that will help you know how to choose the right supplements.
• Free, yet effective ways to get relief from arthritis pain and

inflammation, so you don't have to suffer anymore.
the effects arthritis can have significant impact on your physical and mental well-being, but this books shows you how to overcome its painful symptoms and live life relatively pain free.

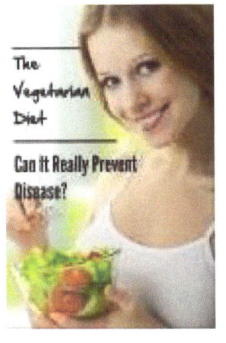

The Vegetarian Diet – Can It Really Prevent Disease?

https://www.createspace.com/5519874

Is a vegetarian diet right for you? Multiple studies have shown over and over that a vegetarian diet goes along way in preventing certain chronic diseases, such as:

• Heart Disease
• Cancer
• Diverticulitis
• Type 2 Diabetes
• Hypertension
• Obesity
• Kidney Failure

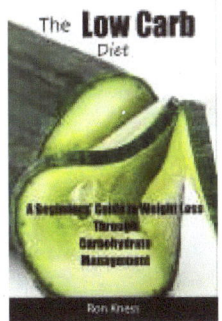

The Low Carb Diet: A Beginner's Guide to Weight Loss Through Carbohydrate Management

https://www.createspace.com/5416348

In my book "The Low-Carb Diet – A

Beginners' Guide to Weight Loss Through Carbohydrate Management", I reveal a successful method of losing weight based in part on the amount and type of carbohydrates you consume.

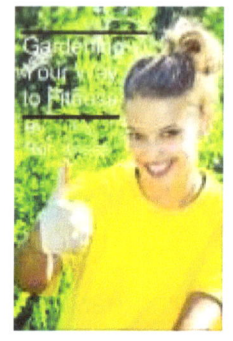

[Gardening Your Way to Fitness: The Fun Way to Get Fit and Provide Beauty and Healthful Bounty for Your Family](https://www.createspace.com/5459564)

https://www.createspace.com/5459564

The gym is a great place to stay fit during the colder seasons, but once the temperature turns warmer you want to spend more time outside. Plus, you'll have the benefit of fresh wholesome produce to enjoy by growing vegetables in your backyard garden.

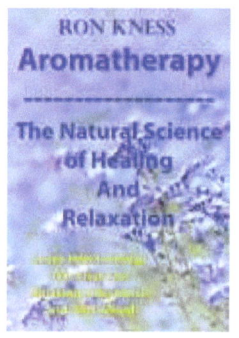

[Aromatherapy - The Science of Healing and Relaxation: Learn How Essential Oils Elicit The Relaxation Response And Alter Mood](https://www.createspace.com/5714434)

https://www.createspace.com/5714434

In my book Aromatherapy – The Science of Healing and Relaxation, we reveal the natural holistics methods you can use to heal the body from certain medical issues and to relive stress through relaxation. In particular we talk about:
• Aromatherapy - what it is and how it works
• Essential Oils – how the effects of certain aromas differs

from others
• Recipes – how to make your own essential oil combinations

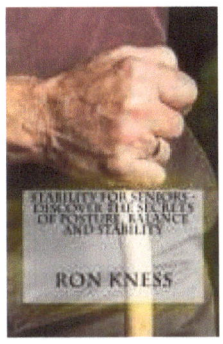

Stability for Seniors: Discover the Secrets of Posture, Balance and Stability

https://www.createspace.com/6096479

Many people sacrifice their health in pursuit of their career. They are so busy making a living that they neglect to make a life. The excuse that they do not have time to exercise is tossed about so frequently that they end up letting their health and fitness slide.

If you are not regularly active, you will have muscular atrophy over time. Your flexibility will decrease. Your core strength will diminish. As time progresses, you will be less limber and more rigid.

This is exactly how people age poorly. It's a process that has snowballed over time.

Only with regular exercise and a healthy diet can you have a body that is fit and has the ability to almost reverse aging.

If you have neglected your health for years and life seems to be a chore now because you can't get around without assistance, do not feel dejected.

You can remedy the situation. You can restore the strength, balance and stamina that you have lost. It is never too late to become what you might have been.

This guide will show you exactly what you need to do to restore your balance, strengthen your core and give you the ability to live life to its fullest. Read how …

About the Author

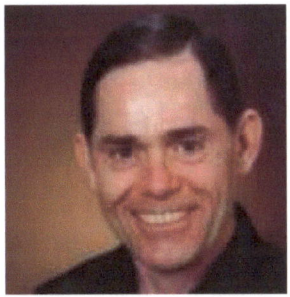

I grew up in Central Minnesota, where my parents owned and operated a fishing resort. Once out of high school I tried a couple of semesters of college, only to quit halfway through the Spring term; I decided at that time that college wasn't for me.

Then I decided to follow my father's previous occupation as an auto mechanic. I graduated from a two-year of vocational training course and worked as a mechanic for five years. While in vocational training, I decided to join the National Guard where I eventually ended up working full-time for 32 years.

So how does all of this relate to writing? In one of my leadership schools, the instructor, who was an English teacher at a juvenile detention center, presented writing to me in a whole new way - a way that started to develop my interest in working with words.

I eventually went back to college on the GI Bill while I was working and earned my Bachelor's degree in Business Administration. Taking a class or two per semester at night and on weekends took me seven years to complete my degree.

Fast forward about 40 years and I now have published over 75 books on Amazon for Kindle, CreateSpace and other publishing platforms.

Besides my own writing, I also ghostwrite ebooks, reports, articles, blogs and do Kindle conversions for clients on a variety of topics.

Today my wife and I are retired from our careers and live in Gold Canyon, AZ. I now write as a retirement business where you'll find me happily sitting in my office typing away on my laptop as I work on my next book or ghostwriting project . . . that is if we are not traveling on a cruise ship - our new-found mode of travel.

www.ingramcontent.com/pod-product-compliance
Lightning Source LLC
Chambersburg PA
CBHW050824290526
45792CB00001B/246